CLINIC CONSULT
PEDIATRICS

Typhoid

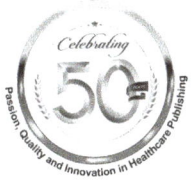

CLINIC CONSULT
PEDIATRICS

Typhoid

Authors

Jaydeep Choudhury DNB (Ped) MNAMS FIAP
Professor
Department of Pediatrics
Institute of Child Health
Kolkata, West Bengal, India

Ritabrata Kundu MD (Ped) FIAP
Professor
Department of Pediatrics
Institute of Child Health
Kolkata, West Bengal, India

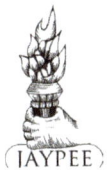

JAYPEE BROTHERS MEDICAL PUBLISHERS
The Health Sciences Publisher
New Delhi | London

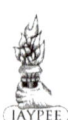

Jaypee Brothers Medical Publishers (P) Ltd

Headquarters
Jaypee Brothers Medical Publishers (P) Ltd
4838/24, Ansari Road, Daryaganj
New Delhi 110 002, India
Phone: +91-11-43574357
Fax: +91-11-43574314
Email: jaypee@jaypeebrothers.com

Overseas Offices
J.P. Medical Ltd
83 Victoria Street, London
SW1H 0HW (UK)
Phone: +44 20 3170 8910
Fax: +44 (0)20 3008 6180
Email: info@jpmedpub.com

Website: www.jaypeebrothers.com
Website: www.jaypeedigital.com

© 2020, Jaypee Brothers Medical Publishers

The views and opinions expressed in this book are solely those of the original contributor(s)/author(s) and do not necessarily represent those of editor(s) of the book.

All rights reserved. No part of this publication may be reproduced, stored or transmitted in any form or by any means, electronic, mechanical, photocopying, recording or otherwise, without the prior permission in writing of the publishers.

All brand names and product names used in this book are trade names, service marks, trademarks or registered trademarks of their respective owners. The publisher is not associated with any product or vendor mentioned in this book.

Medical knowledge and practice change constantly. This book is designed to provide accurate, authoritative information about the subject matter in question. However, readers are advised to check the most current information available on procedures included and check information from the manufacturer of each product to be administered, to verify the recommended dose, formula, method and duration of administration, adverse effects and contraindications. It is the responsibility of the practitioner to take all appropriate safety precautions. Neither the publisher nor the author(s)/editor(s) assume any liability for any injury and/or damage to persons or property arising from or related to use of material in this book.

This book is sold on the understanding that the publisher is not engaged in providing professional medical services. If such advice or services are required, the services of a competent medical professional should be sought.

Every effort has been made where necessary to contact holders of copyright to obtain permission to reproduce copyright material. If any have been inadvertently overlooked, the publisher will be pleased to make the necessary arrangements at the first opportunity. The **CD/DVD-ROM** (if any) provided in the sealed envelope with this book is complimentary and free of cost. **Not meant for sale.**

Inquiries for bulk sales may be solicited at: jaypee@jaypeebrothers.com

Clinic Consult Pediatrics: Typhoid / Jaydeep Choudhury, Ritabrata Kundu

First Edition: 2020

ISBN: 978-93-5270-707-2

Dedicated to
Our Students
*A constant encouragement for
our academic endeavors*

Preface

Typhoid is one of the most common infectious diseases in the Indian subcontinent. The typical presentation is fever, but it has a wide range of manifestations and some children may require hospital admission.

Southeast Asia, South-central Asia and parts of Africa reports high incidence of *Salmonella typhi* infection, accounting for more than 100 cases per 100,000 person-years. *Salmonella paratyphi* also accounts for a substantial proportion of enteric fever cases in areas of South Asia but it remains uncommon in Africa. Lack of consistent reporting from different areas of the world is the main limitation for getting a true picture of global scenario.

Humans are the only reservoir for *S. typhi* but a specific source or contact is identified only in a small number of cases. A typhoid case or carrier is the source of infection but often unnoticed.

Specific diagnosis of an infectious disease like typhoid has several advantages. It helps in reducing the financial expense considerably. Prompt and appropriate antimicrobial therapy can be initiated, which ensures prevention of antimicrobial resistance. The threat of extensively drug-resistant typhoid (XDR typhoid) is looming on the horizon; our neighboring country Pakistan has reported good number of cases. Proper preventive measures can help to reduce the disease burden in a large way.

It is needless to say that a good microbiology laboratory is vital in the isolation and identification of organisms including resistance pattern.

Monotherapy is still the thumb rule for antibiotic treatment of typhoid fever. Antibiotics in appropriate doses ensure good response and prevent further complications. It is heartening to note that typhoid is again becoming susceptible to the first-line antibiotics, though their routine use is not recommended at present. The cost of treating typhoid has escalated with the use of third-generation cephalosporins. Rampant indiscriminate use of azithromycin will make this easily available cheap drug useless in the coming years. It is important that azithromycin is used judiciously.

Environmental protection is one of the vital issues in prevention of typhoid in the community level. It is imperative that mass scale sanitary and personal hygiene improvement is a difficult proposition. Vaccination against typhoid is an important preventive strategy on an individual basis.

The chapters compiled in this book cover the various aspects of typhoid in a concise easy to read presentation. This book is meant for all the medical practitioners who treat patients suffering from typhoid and also for undergraduate and postgraduate medical students.

Jaydeep Choudhury
Ritabrata Kundu

Acknowledgment

We are deeply indebted to the innumerable patients suffering from typhoid who attend our hospital. They have taught us the most.

We would like to express our gratitude to Professor Apurba Ghosh and Professor Maya Mukhopadhyay for always being kind and supportive to us for all our endeavors. Whenever we undertake any academic project we remember Late Dr Tapan Kumar Ghosh who has influenced our lives in many ways.

Our honest appreciation for Mr Somnath Mukherjee and Ms Ruma Saha for secretarial assistance during preparation of the manuscript.

Sincere gratitude to our family members for being supportive to us.

We appreciate the support and cooperation that we have always received from Shri Jitender P Vij (Chairman and Managing Director), Mr Ankit Vij, Mr Shashi Kumar Sambhoo, Dr Neeraj Choudhary, Ms Sudarshna Agarwal, Mrs Samina Khan and the team of M/s Jaypee Brothers Medical Publishers (P) Ltd, New Delhi and Mr Sandeep Gupta, Mr Sabyasachi Hazra and the team from Kolkata Branch for their wholehearted effort and cooperation.

Contents

CHAPTER 1
Epidemiology — 1

CHAPTER 2
Pathogenesis — 7

CHAPTER 3
Clinical Features — 14

CHAPTER 4
Complications — 19

CHAPTER 5
Investigations — 27

CHAPTER 6
Treatment — 38

CHAPTER 7
Prevention — 48

CHAPTER 8
Vaccines — 51

CHAPTER 1

Epidemiology

INTRODUCTION

Typhoid fever is endemic in many developing countries due to poor sanitation and contaminated water supply. It is caused due to infection by the genus *Salmonella* which comprises of *Salmonella typhi*, *S. paratyphi A*, *S. paratyphi B* and *S. paratyphi C*. All these organisms can cause a bacteremic illness known as enteric fever. Among all these, *S. typhi* causes typhoid fever and the rest causes paratyphoid fever. Human is the only reservoir in the form of either cases or carriers. Infected patients excrete these organisms for varying periods of times. Those patients who excrete *S. typhi* bacilli for more than 1 year after clinical or subclinical typhoid infection are classified as chronic carriers. Nearly 3–5% of the typhoid fever cases become chronic carriers.

EPIDEMIOLOGY

The regional typhoid fever rates are classified as high (>100 cases/100,000/year), medium (10–100 cases/100,000/year), and low (<10 cases/100,000/year) incidence settings. India including South Central Asia has an incidence setting of roughly 622 cases/100,000/year suggesting to be in high incidence setting group.[1] Community-based studies show consistently higher levels of typhoid than public health figure. Annual incidence rate of 980/100,000 in Delhi has been reported from our country.[2]

Typhoid fever may occur at any age but it is more prevalent in children and young adults, the peak incidence is in children aged 5–15 years. As the person grows older he becomes relatively immune because of the acquired immunity due to subclinical exposure to typhoid bacilli. Cases occur throughout the year but increase during the summers, the peak months being July to September.

CAUSATIVE ORGANISM

Salmonella is a gram negative bacillus. The organism survives intracellularly, grows rapidly on ordinary media under aerobic as well as anaerobic conditions. It is rapidly killed by drying, pasteurization and common disinfectants. *S. typhi*, *S. paratyphi A*, *S. paratyphi B* and *S. paratyphi C* organisms have three main antigens O, H and Vi. *S. typhi* has more than 80 phage types. Phage typing is a useful epidemiological tool in tracing the source of epidemics. *S. typhi* and *paratyphi* together form a group of fever referred to as enteric fever. Typhoid contributes 90% in this group.

Salmonella survive refrigeration and also heating. They may remain viable at ambient temperatures and also in various foods for weeks. It may remain viable in foods after low heat cooking (less than 140°C) cooked for less than 12 minutes. *Salmonella* may survive for hours in the hand of food handlers.[3]

INCUBATION PERIOD

Incubation period of *Salmonella* is 10–14 days. It may be as short as 3 days and as long as 3 weeks. It depends on the load of the bacillus ingested. The incubation period is inversely proportional to the size of inoculum. *S. typhi* divides rapidly in less than half hour. So that, after 1–2 weeks, the amount of bacilli that results from even a single bacillus are tremendous. Thus, the total bacilli load is usually huge. However, normal intestinal flora is an important defense against invasion by typhoid bacillus and not all persons who get infected would get the disease eventually.

SOURCE OF INFECTION

The primary source of infection is the feces and urine of cases and carriers. The secondary sources are contaminated water, food, and dissemination by hands and flies. *S. typhi* does not multiply in water but can survive for about a week. In soil irrigated with water from sewage, *S. typhi* may survive for nearly 2 months. It can survive for more than a month in ice and ice-creams. *S. typhi* can also grow rapidly in milk without altering its taste or appearance. Milk products like cream, ice-cream and cheese have also been known to have caused *Salmonella* epidemics. Vegetables grown on sewage irrigated farms may be infected with typhoid bacilli and can be a source of infection if taken raw without being washed properly or disinfecting them by using chlorine and potassium permanganate. Other food sources which can commonly lead to infection are meat products (when not cooked well) and untreated shellfish. The organism remains viable on external surface of houseflies for as long as 20 days. These flies carry the bacillus from the feces to food and are thus an important source of infection.[4]

Various personal and social factors or practices which are conducive for the spread of infection are improper hand washing after toilets, low standard of food and kitchen hygiene, washing infected material near kitchen, defecation and urination in open spaces, illiteracy and lack of health education. Inadequate facilities for processing human waste further contaminates water supply. Patients with parasitic infections such as roundworms or schistosomiasis are also readily infected with *S. typhi* as the organism gets adhered to the surface of the parasites.

EPIDEMIOLOGY OF MULTIDRUG RESISTANT TYPHOID FEVER

Multiple drug resistant *S. typhi* (MDRST) denotes those strains of typhoid fever which have resistance to all the three first line antibiotics (chloramphenicol, ampicillin and trimethoprim/sulfamethoxazole). It has assumed a massive proportion not only in many developing countries but is also being increasingly seen in the developed countries.[3]

Initially in 1948 chloramphenicol was the treatment of choice for typhoid. It was in 1972 that major resistance to this drug developed and outbreaks occurred in many countries including India. Toward the end of 1990s typhoid was resistant to all the first-line drugs and infections with these strains were reported from India also.[5]

Fluoroquinolones was the next drug to be introduced in the treatment of typhoid but resistance to this drug was also reported. So, there are two categories of drug resistance—resistance to first-line antibiotics and resistance to the fluoroquinolone drugs. Resistance to fluoroquinolone may again be total or partial. The so called nalidixic acid resistant *S. typhi* (NARST) is a marker of reduced susceptibility to fluoroquinolones compared to nalidixic acid sensitive strains. Nalidixic acid is not used for the treatment of typhoid. NARST isolates are susceptible to fluoroquinolones in current disk sensitivity test. But the clinical response to treatment with fluoroquinolones of NARST is worse than with nalidixic acid sensitive strains.[6,7] This reduced susceptibility to fluoroquinolones has become a major problem in Asia.

Third generation cephalosporins including oral cefixime and parenteral ceftriaxone were found to be effective in children.[3] Sporadic reports of high level resistance to ceftriaxone followed though rare. Recently, azithromycin is used in children for the treatment of uncomplicated typhoid fever.

KEY MESSAGES

- Poor sanitation and contaminated water supply are the main causes of endemicity of typhoid in developing countries
- Human is the only reservoir of typhoid
- India including South Central Asia falls into the high incidence setting group of typhoid
- *Salmonella* survive refrigeration, heating including low heat cooking, stored food for weeks and also for hours in the hand of food handlers
- The source of infection primarily is feces and urine of cases and carriers and secondarily by contaminated water, food and dissemination by hands and flies.

REFERENCES

1. Crump JA, Luby SP, Mintz ED. The global burden of typhoid fever. Bull WHO 2004;82:346-53.
2. Sinha A, Sazawal S, Kumar R, et al. Typhoid fever in children aged less than 5 years. Lancet 1999;354:734-7.
3. Ochoa TJ, Santisteban Ponce J. *Salmonella*. In: Cherry JD, Steinbach WJ, Harrison GJ, Hotez PJ, Kaplan SL, editors. Feigin and Cherry's Textbook of Pediatric Infectious Diseases, 8th edition. Philadelphia: Elsevier, 2019;1066-80.

4. Parry CM, Hien TT, Dougan G, White NJ, Farrar JJ. Typhoid Fever. N Engl J Med 2002;347:1770-82.
5. Bhutta ZA. Impact of age and drug resistance on mortality in typhoid fever. Arch Dis Child 1996;75:214-7.
6. Crump JA, Barrett TJ, Nelson JT, Angulo FJ. Reevaluating fluoroquinolone breakpoints for *Salmonella enterica* serotype typhi and for non-typhi salmonellae. Clin Infect Dis 2003;37:75-81.
7. Kapil A, Das B. Nalidixic acid susceptibility test to screen ciprofloxacin resistance in *Salmonella typhi*. Indian J Med Res 2002;115:49-54.

CHAPTER 2

Pathogenesis

INTRODUCTION

The invasiveness of *Salmonella* is regulated by growth state, high osmolarity, low oxygen tension and pH. *Salmonella typhi* must survive the gastric acid barrier to reach the small intestine and a low gastric pH is an important defense mechanism. The infectious dose of *S. typhi* in volunteers varies between 1,000 and 1 million organisms. Vi-negative strains of *S. typhi* are less infectious and less virulent than Vi-positive strains.[1]

Increased susceptibility to *Salmonella* is seen in conditions that decrease stomach acidity (children below 1 year age, antacid ingestion and achlorhydria) and in conditions that decrease intestinal integrity (inflammatory bowel disease, gastrointestinal surgery, alteration of intestinal flora by antibiotic administration). Flowchart 1 shows the pathogenic mechanism of typhoid.

IN THE SMALL INTESTINE

The bacteria reach the small intestine where they colonize. It then adheres to the intestinal epithelia via five different fimbrial operons (fim, lpf, agf, sef and pef). Lpf are important in the initial attachment to Peyer's patches. These are lymphoid follicles similar in many ways to lymph nodes, located in

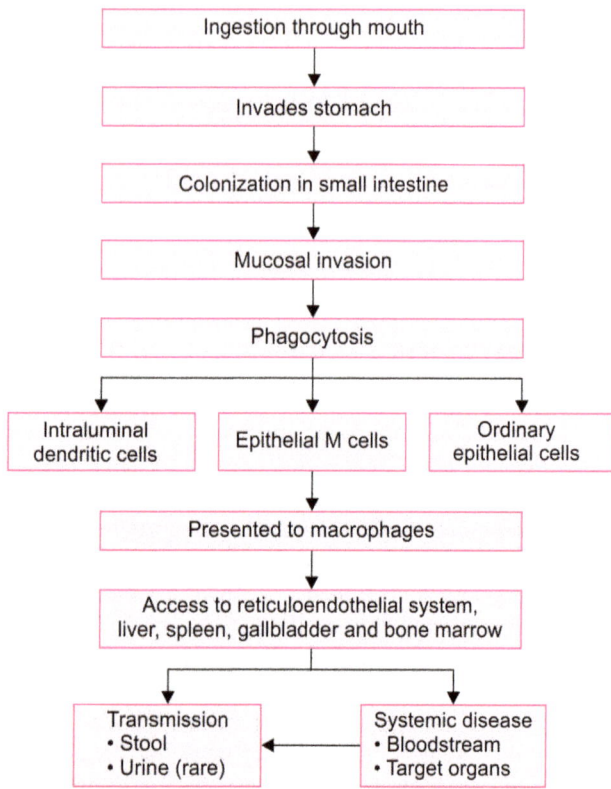

FLOWCHART 1: Pathogenetic mechanism for typhoid.

the mucosa and extending into the submucosa of small intestine. It is usually found in the lowest portion of the small intestine, mainly in the distal jejunum and the ileum. It could also be detected in the duodenum. In adults, B lymphocytes predominate in Peyer's patches.

Salmonella enter the intestines through phagocytic microfold or M cells overlying the Peyer's patches in small intestine.

Pathogenesis

These M Cells, specialized epithelial cells overlying Peyer's patches, are probably the site of the internalization of *S. typhi*.

Salmonella also enter nonphagocytic epithelial cells by a process known as bacteria-mediated endocytosis. This is thought to be facilitated by direct translocation of *Salmonella* proteins into the host cell cytoplasm by a specialized secretion apparatus (type III secretion). This mechanism promotes survival of bacteria within the phagocytes. The easy access through the bowel may be explained by the bacteria's ability to invade the gut without stimulating an acute inflammatory response or recruitment of neutrophils.

IN THE BLOOD STREAM

After passing through the intestinal epithelial cells, they reach the lamina propria where they are phagocytosed by macrophages. The bacteria are conveyed to the draining mesenteric lymph nodes and from there reach the blood stream via the thoracic duct. This transient primary bacteremia is followed by seeding of the reticuloendothelial cells of different organs like liver, spleen and bone morrow.

BACTEREMIA

During the incubation period, the organisms multiply silently within sites to which they have been seeded by the primary bacteremia. The onset of symptoms correlates with the secondary persistent bacteremia into the blood of large number of organisms from primarily infected sites. The gallbladder is particularly susceptible to being infected and constantly delivers more bacilli to the intestine via the bile.

The surface Vi capsular antigen interferes with phagocytosis by preventing the binding of C3 to the surface of bacterium. The ability of bacteria to survive within macrophages after phagocytosis is an important virulence trait encoded by the PhoP regulon.

Circulating endotoxin, a lipopolysaccharide component of bacterial cell wall is thought to cause the prolonged fever and toxic symptoms of enteric fever, although its levels in symptomatic patients are often low. Alternatively, endotoxin-induced cytokine production by macrophages when a critical number of organisms have replicated may cause systemic symptoms. At a critical point that is probably determined by the number of bacteria, their virulence, and the host response, bacteria are released from this sequestered intracellular habitat into the bloodstream.[1]

ORGAN INVOLVEMENT

In the bacteremic phase, the organism is widely disseminated throughout the body. The most common sites of secondary infection are the liver, spleen, bone marrow, gallbladder and Peyer's patches of the terminal ileum.[2] Gallbladder invasion occurs either directly from the blood or by retrograde spread from the bile. Organisms excreted in the bile either reinvade the intestinal wall or are excreted in the feces. Proliferation of bacilli, which is enhanced by bile, continues in the bile ducts and especially in the gallbladder, from where large numbers of bacteria pass into the gut and may be cultured from a duodenal aspirate.

After the macrophages have been activated by sensitized lymphocytes, an inflammatory reaction takes place and results in swelling, necrosis and ulceration of Peyer's patches, which in most cases, heals uneventfully.[3]

The hepatosplenomegaly is due to recruitment of mononuclear cells and the development of a cell-mediated immune response to *S. typhi* colonization. The recruitment of additional mononuclear cells and lymphocytes Peyer's patches afterwards can result in marked enlargement of Peyer's patches, with right lower quadrant abdominal pain. However, erosion of blood vessels may cause intestinal hemorrhage and extension of necrosis through the bowel wall may result in perforation.

Many tissues of the body can be affected, including liver, spleen, kidney, heart and lungs.

Typhoid nodules, which are foci of macrophages and lymphocytes, can be detected in a large number of internal organs.

NEUROPSYCHIATRIC COMPLICATIONS

Various neuropsychiatric complications are common in typhoid fever. The exact pathogenesis is not known. However, various mechanisms have been postulated.[3]

- Endotoxin as well as bacteria (*Salmonella*) per se may produce myelitis
- Nonspecific allergic demyelinating form of encephalomyelitis which may occur as a reaction to a number of bacterial and viral illnesses
- An "endarteritis obliterans" producing thrombosis and ultimate paraplegia.

Pathological changes in patients with neuropsychiatric complications reveals varying lesions such as diffuse neuronal damage, nonspecific vascular changes with thrombosis and hemorrhages, perivascular softening, and disseminated granuloma formation.

MECHANISMS OF IMMUNITY

Cell-mediated immunity is probably the key factor in production of immunity and recovery from infection. Humoral antibody production appears to play minimal role in recovery from acute infection, as the patient continues to deteriorate despite the appearance of O, H and Vi antibodies.[4]

Local gut immunity, both innate and acquired is also important in preventing infection and re-infection.

In endemic countries, typhoid fever has highest prevalence in children and adolescents.[1] Adults are protected after having acquired substantial immunity to previous subclinical exposures.

KEY MESSAGES

- Invasiveness of *Salmonella* is regulated by growth state of the bacteria, high osmolarity, low oxygen tension, high pH, inflammatory bowel disease, gastrointestinal surgery and alteration of intestinal flora by antibiotic use
- The bacteria adhere to the epithelium of small intestine then they are conveyed to the draining mesenteric lymph nodes and reach the blood stream via the thoracic duct. Finally seed the reticuloendothelial cells of liver, spleen and bone morrow
- Onset of symptoms correlates with the secondary persistent bacteremia from primarily infected sites
- The organism is widely disseminated in liver, spleen, bone marrow, gallbladder and Peyer's patches of the terminal ileum
- Gallbladder is invaded either directly from the blood or by retrograde spread from the bile.

REFERENCES

1. Ochoa TJ, Santisteban Ponce J. *Salmonella*. In: Cherry JD, Steinbach WJ, Harrison GJ, Hotez PJ, Kaplan SL, editors. Feigin and Cherry's Textbook of Pediatric Infectious Diseases, 8th edition. Philadelphia: Elsevier, 2019;1066-80.

2. Richens J. Typhoid fever. In: Cohen J, Powderly WG, editors. Infectious diseases, 2nd edition. London: Harcourt Publishers Ltd, 2004:1561.
3. McKinney JS. Enteric fever (Typhoid fever). In: Kliegman RM, Blum NJ, Shah SS, St Geme JW, Tasker RC, Walson KM. Nelson Textbook of Pediatrics, 21st edition. Philadelphia: Elsevier, 2020;1502-7.
4. Parry CM, Hien TT, Dougan G, White NJ, Farrar JJ. Typhoid fever. N Engl J Med 2002;347:1770-82.

CHAPTER 3

Clinical Features

INTRODUCTION

The classical features of typhoid fever are mainly found in school-age children and young adults. Infants and young children often have atypical presentation. The clinical features vary with the age group, from patient to patient and in geographical locations.[1] The disease often does not have any definite distinguishing feature and the diagnosis is sometimes made after several days by exclusion.

The clinical features of typhoid fever usually manifest in children toward the end of the first week or second week after the infection. The typical features at the onset are fever, chills, malaise, anorexia, nausea, poorly localized abdominal discomfort, a dry cough and myalgia. At this stage, there are hardly any physical signs. In the later phase of illness a child may present with signs of toxicity. The tongue may be coated. Diffuse tenderness in abdomen with hepatomegaly and splenomegaly are common in this phase.[2] The disease often has no characteristic distinguishing features. Thus, diagnosis is sometimes made after several days and by process of exclusion.

FEVER

Fever is the most constant presentation of typhoid fever and is present in all patients.[1] The onset of fever is gradual and the patients may find it difficult to recollect when exactly the fever started. Initially, the fever is low grade, but it rises progressively, in a stepwise fashion and by the second week it is often high and sustained at 39–40°C (102–104°F). This typical pattern may not be found always, instead if there is fever without focus for more than 4 days duration one should consider enteric fever. In most cases, there is no definite pattern of fever. The step ladder patterns of fever mentioned are relics of preantibiotic era and are not seen these days. Some children may have accompanying chills and rigor. Older children may complain of body ache, headache and anorexia.

GASTROINTESTINAL MANIFESTATIONS

Gastrointestinal manifestations are often seen in typhoid fever. Among these, the most common presentations are abdominal pain, splenohepatomegaly, anorexia, vomiting and diarrhea.[3] A soft spleen becomes palpable under the costal margin at the end of the first week. Splenomegaly is present in about 60% and hepatomegaly in about 40% patients of typhoid fever. Hepatomegaly is more common in children below 2 years. Abdominal symptoms including distension, tenderness, cecal gurgling (typhlitis), tympanitic abdomen and disturbance of bowel movement are sometimes seen in children.[4]

Diarrhea is common in typhoid fever. The stool may be watery but usually does not cause dehydration. Stool may be foul smelling and thicker, referred as pea soup stool.[5] Diarrhea generally starts 3 days after the onset of fever and lasts for a few days. Constipation is more likely in older children later course of disease.

CARDIORESPIRATORY MANIFESTATIONS

The respiratory rate is often raised and nonlocalized rhonchi and crepitations may be heard. A relative bradycardia may be found in late stage in older children. Signs of heart failure may be present, though rarely, if there is anemia or myocarditis.

SKIN MANIFESTATIONS

Rose spots, typically blanching erythematous maculopapular lesions approximately 2–4 mm in diameter, are reported in 5–30% of cases.[2] It is not easily seen in Indian children. They usually occur on the abdomen and chest and rarely on the back, arms and legs. They leave a slightly brownish discoloration of the skin on healing.

OTHER MANIFESTATIONS

During the second week of illness, high fever is sustained and prostrations, fatigue, anorexia, cough and abdominal symptoms increase in severity. Inflammation may be observed in the form of cholecystitis, localized abscesses, pneumonia, bronchitis, septic arthritis, osteomyelitis, pyelonephritis, endophthalmitis and meningitis. Glomerulonephritis may occur in some cases due to immune complex disease.[5] *S. typhi* osteomyelitis is commonly associated with sickle cell disease. Patients may appear acutely ill, disoriented and lethargic. Delirium and stupor may be observed. Meningism may be seen in some children.[2] Many patients may have a characteristic apathetic affect (coma vigil). In infants and young children, the disease is often mild at presentation, mimicking a viral prodrome.[3]

DIFFERENTIAL DIAGNOSIS

Malaria

The constellation of features like high fever with chills and rigors, splenohepatomegaly often mimics malaria. But contrary to the manifestation in typhoid infection, fever is usually of abrupt onset in malaria.

Viral Hepatitis

Reduced appetite, fever and hepatomegaly may be the initial presentation of viral hepatitis. Although jaundice is not common in typhoid fever, but it may occur in some children and liver function tests may be deranged.

Pneumonia

The presentation of fever, cough and chest findings may mimic pneumonia. Presence of associated abdominal findings indicates typhoid fever.

Typhoid fever has to be differentiated from various acute and subacute febrile illnesses. Tuberculosis, liver abscess, other deep abscesses, leptospirosis, infectious mononucleosis, infective endocarditis and connective tissue disorders could be the other differential diagnosis.

KEY MESSAGES

- ❏ The clinical features of typhoid fever usually manifest in children toward the end of the first week or second week after the infection
- ❏ Fever is the most constant presentation of typhoid fever

- ❏ The most common gastrointestinal manifestations are abdominal pain, hepatosplenomegaly, anorexia, vomiting and diarrhea
- ❏ A toxic child with coated tongue, tender abdomen, hepatomegaly and splenomegaly are common in the later phase of illness
- ❏ Typhoid often does not have any definite distinguishing feature and diagnosis is sometimes made by exclusion.

REFERENCES

1. Ochoa TJ, Santisteban Ponce J. *Salmonella*. In: Cherry JD, Steinbach WJ, Harrison GJ, Hotez PJ, Kaplan SL, editors. Feigin and Cherry's Textbook of Pediatric Infectious Diseases, 8th edition. Philadelphia: Elsevier, 2019;1066-80.
2. McKinney JS. Enteric fever (Typhoid fever). In: Kliegman RM, Blum NJ, Shah SS, St Geme JW, Tasker RC, Walson KM. Nelson Textbook of Pediatrics, 21st edition. Philadelphia: Elsevier, 2020;1502-7.
3. Choudhury J, Kundu R. Enteric fever. In: Choudhury J, Kundu R, editors. Pediatric Infectious Diseases, 1st edition. New Delhi: Jaypee Brothers, 2012;308-20.
4. Garg RA, Krashak R. Typhoid fever before two years of age. Indian Pediatr 1993;30:805-8.
5. Roy K, Kundu R. Typhoid fever. In: Parthasarathy A, Menon PSN, Nair MKC, et al, editors. IAP Textbook of Pediatrics, 7th edition. New Delhi: Jaypee Brothers, 2019;407-11.

CHAPTER 4

Complications

INTRODUCTION

Typhoid fever is infamous for its myriad complications. Most of the complications of typhoid fever occur after the first week of illness. Complications occur in 10–15% of patients and are particularly likely in children who have been ill for more than 2 weeks.[1] Complications referred to every system of the body have been described. The main complications which endanger life are intestinal perforation and hemorrhage but relapse is a frequent complication which prolongs the illness. Relapse occurs in 5–10% of patients, usually 2–3 weeks after the resolution of fever.[2] Reinfection may also occur and can be distinguished from relapse by molecular typing.

The average case fatality rate is less than 1%. The case fatality rates are highest among children under 1 year of age.[3] However, the most important contributor to a poor outcome is probably a delay in instituting effective antibiotic treatment.[4]

Factors which increase the incidence of complications of typhoid fever are:
- Poor accessibility to healthcare facility
- Lack of early diagnostic facility
- Late initiation of antibiotics
- Inadequate and inappropriate treatment

- Other associated illnesses like malnutrition, HIV infection, innate immunodeficiency and sickle cell disease
- Staying in a community with high incidence of multidrug resistant typhoid is a contributing factor.

SEVERE TYPHOID FEVER

These patients represent an important subgroup of typhoid fever having high mortality rate (50%). It can be identified on the basis of mental state and cardiovascular status. The criteria for severe typhoid are marked mental confusion, delirium, obtundation, stupor or coma, and shock defined by systolic BP less than 80 mm Hg with evidence of decreased skin, cerebral or renal perfusion.[1]

Gastrointestinal Complication

Intestinal Hemorrhage

Intestinal hemorrhage may be seen in the middle of second week due to erosion of a blood vessel by the ulcerating Peyer's patches. It is rare in children under 10 years of age. The bleeding may manifest as frank bleeding or presence of altered blood in stool and it may be slight or massive. It is a self-limiting process and does not need surgery.

Intestinal Perforation

Intestinal perforation is the most feared complication of typhoid fever. It is the leading cause of mortality in children suffering from typhoid fever. Although the incidence is very low, it is responsible for 25% of mortality.[5] It is not related to the severity of disease and it is usually seen in the third week of illness. The usual site of perforation is terminal ilium. The presentation may be acute or subacute. Patients present with severe abdominal pain localized mainly in the right lower quadrant, abdominal guarding, rebound tenderness on palpation and rigidity. Vomiting is almost always present. Occurrence of sudden onset pain along with rise in pulse rate and fall in blood pressure are the characteristic presentation. Free fluid in the abdomen and gas under the diaphragm clinches the diagnosis. Antibiotics form the mainstay of therapy along with conservative management.

Other gastrointestinal manifestations may be paralytic ileus, jaundice, cholecystitis and rarely spontaneous rupture of spleen.

Cardiovascular Complications

The most common cardiovascular complication of typhoid fever is nonspecific electrocardiogram (ECG) changes, it occurs in 10–15% of patients.[2] Various ECG changes are low voltage tracings, depressed ST segments and T wave inversion.
Other complications are:
- *Myocarditis:* It is usually asymptomatic and associated with nonspecific ECG changes. But it may present with chest pain, congestive heart failure, cardiogenic shock, and may cause immediate death
- *Arrhythmias:* Disorders of conduction or even heart block has been described
- *Pericarditis:* It is rare in children
- *Venous thrombosis:* Rare in children. Femoral vein thrombosis may occur in fourth week of illness. It may involve the calf veins. An increase in pulse rate along with fever, swelling and tenderness in calf muscles is the presentation. Arterial thrombosis is less common but more serious.

Pulmonary Complications

- *Bronchitis:* It is quite common in children and manifests as dry cough

- *Lobar pneumonia:* It is usually seen in second week of illness. It should be suspected when pneumonia does not respond to usual antibiotics and *S. typhi* is cultured both from blood and sputum
- *Laryngitis:* It is an occasional late complication due to ulceration of posterior wall of larynx. It presents with hoarse voice, stridor and painful swallowing
- *Hemorrhagic pleural effusion and empyema:* Rare complications.

Neuropsychiatric Complications

Typhoid fever is associated with a variety of neuropsychiatric complications in about 50% of patients. The most frequent complication is disturbance in the level of consciousness. It may range from disorientation, delirium, obtundation, stupor to coma.[5] Of these, delirium is the earliest neurological symptom observed. Post typhoid confusion may persist for weeks to months, but recovery is the rule.

The factors responsible for neurological manifestation of typhoid fever are hyperpyrexia, fluid and electrolyte disturbance, release of typhoid neurotoxin, vasculitis and autoimmune mechanism.

- *Typhoid state (Typhoid encephalopathy):* Commonly found in second week of illness. It is acute toxic confusional state characterized by disorientation, delirium and restlessness. Delirium, stupor and coma are associated with poor prognosis with case fatality rate more than 40%. Delirium, if it persis even after the temperature and metabolic abnormality has returned to normal is associated with worst prognosis
- *Typhoid meningitis:* Usually seen in children less than 5 years of age. It mimics pyogenic meningitis

- *Other rare neurological complications:* Includes seizures, cerebellar ataxia, brain abscess, depression, schizophrenic states with catatonic encephalomyelitis, transverse myelitis, peripheral neuropathy, cranial neuropathy, acute disseminated encephalomyelitis (ADEM) and Guillain-Barré syndrome.[5]

Genitourinary Complications

- *Asymptomatic excretion of S. typhi in urine:* Present in 25% cases in various stages of typhoid fever
- *Transient proteinuria:* This is the most common genitourinary complication. Rarely there may be immune-complex mediated glomerulonephritis presenting as renal failure or nephrotic syndrome
- Suppurative typhoid pyelonephritis
- Cystitis
- Orchitis.

Hepatobiliary Complications

- *Typhoid hepatitis:* It may result in asymptomatic elevation of liver enzymes
- *Jaundice:* It is due to hepatitis, cholecystitis or hemolytic anemia
- Acute cholecystitis
- Chronic cholecystitis.

Hematological Complications

Hemolytic anemia: Anemia is almost universal in children suffering from typhoid fever, especially in children below 2 years of age. The various causes for anemia may be hemolysis, bone marrow suppression, intestinal hemorrhage or disseminated intravascular coagulation (DIC). Hemolytic-uremic syndrome with mild form of DIC has also been described.[1]

Leukopenia with neutropenia and relative lymphocytosis is a common finding. Lymphopenia is more common, present in 75%.

Musculoskeletal Complications

- *Periostitis:* Commonly involves tibia and ribs
- *Arthritis:* It usually involves hips, knee and ankle
- *Zenker's degeneration of muscles:* Abdominal wall muscles and thighs
- Polymyositis.

Others

Parotitis and typhoid abscess. Due to sustained bacteremia, focal infection can develop at any site. The common sites are bone, brain, liver, spleen, etc.

RELAPSE

Salmonella typhi displays an unusual affinity to stay inside the body and relapse with an intervening normal period described as short as 1 day to as long as 70 days.[2] It manifests clinically by a recurrence of fever and other symptoms. Fever generally reappears about 2 weeks after the completion of antibiotic therapy.[1] But relapse may occur during convalescence, when the child is afebrile, asymptomatic but on antibiotic. It may occur several months after the initial infection also. Rarely a chronic relapsing form has been found lasting for many months especially after treatment with insufficient doses of antibiotics. Relapses are usually milder. Relapse typhoid fever is diagnosed when the clinical symptoms reappear along with culture positive infection with an antibiogram similar to the initial isolate within 8 weeks of completion of successful therapy of initial infection. In spite of appropriate therapy, 2–4% of infected children may experience relapse after initial response to treatment. Relapse typhoid fever should be treated with the same antibiotics with proper dose and duration.[4] Multiple recurrences of septicemic *Salmonella* with metastatic foci may occur in association with sickle cell disease and HIV infection.

KEY MESSAGES

- Most of the complications of typhoid fever occur after the first week of illness
- Criteria for severe typhoid are mental confusion, delirium, obtundation, stupor or coma, shock with evidence of decreased skin, cerebral or renal perfusion
- Intestinal hemorrhage and perforation are the common gastrointestinal complications
- Most common cardiovascular complication of typhoid fever is nonspecific ECG changes
- Dry cough due to bronchitis is common in children
- Neuropsychiatric complications may be present in about 50% of patients; the most frequent complication is disturbance in the level of consciousness
- Anemia is almost universal in children suffering from typhoid fever
- Typhoid hepatitis, jaundice, acute or chronic cholecystitis are the hepatobiliary complications
- Asymptomatic bacteriuria, transient proteinuris, cystitis are urinary complications
- Typhoid relapse with appearance of fever after an intervening normal period may be seen.

REFERENCES

1. Choudhury J, Kundu R. Enteric fever. In: Choudhury J, Kundu R, editors. Pediatric Infectious Diseases, 1st edition. New Delhi: Jaypee Brothers, 2012;308-20.
2. Ochoa TJ, Santisteban Ponce J. *Salmonella*. In: Cherry JD, Steinbach WJ, Harrison GJ, Hotez PJ, Kaplan SL, editors. Feigin and Cherry's Textbook of Pediatric Infectious Diseases, 8th edition. Philadelphia: Elsevier, 2019;1066-80.
3. Parry CM, Hien TT, Dougan G, White NJ, Farrar JJ. Typhoid fever. N Engl J Med 2002;347:1770-82.
4. Shastri D, Singhal T. Antimicrobial therapy in enteric fever. In: Singhal T, Shah N, Prabhu S, Yewale V, editors, 3rd edition. New Delhi: Jaypee Brothers, 2019;252-9.
5. McKinney JS. Enteric fever (Typhoid fever). In: Kliegman RM, Blum NJ, Shah SS, St Geme JW, Tasker RC, Walson KM. Nelson Textbook of Pediatrics, 21st edition. Philadelphia: Elsevier, 2020;1502-7.

CHAPTER 5

Investigations

INTRODUCTION

Appropriate diagnosis of typhoid is the first and vital step for starting effective therapy. Various investigations should be judged by their use and limitations.

COMPLETE BLOOD COUNT

Complete blood count (CBC) in typhoid is usually unremarkable. The hemoglobin level decreases with disease progression. Severe anemia is uncommon in typhoid and if present it should raise the suspicion of intestinal hemorrhage or hemolysis.[1] The white blood cell count is usually normal in most cases of typhoid fever and leukocytosis makes the diagnosis less likely. Leukopenia may be seen in about 20–25% cases. The differential count is usually unremarkable. Eosinopenia may be present in 70–80% cases, sometimes there may be zero eosinophil count. Platelet counts are usually normal initially and fall in some patients by the second week of illness. Generally, the prevalence of thrombocytopenia is around 10–15%.[2]

CULTURES

Blood Cultures

Blood cultures is the gold standard diagnostic tool for typhoid.[2] Blood culture is most sensitive in the first week of fever when it is about 90% positive and reduces with advancing illness to 40% by fourth week. Overall, the sensitivity of blood culture is around 50% but the sensitivity drops considerably with prior antibiotic therapy.[1]

Causes of failure to isolate the organism by blood culture:
- Inadequate culture media
- Low volume of blood taken and inoculated for culture
- Prior antibiotic therapy
- Time of blood collection.

Salmonella is easy to grow and can be readily cultured in routine culture media like Hartley's media, Blood agar, and MacConkey agar.[1] Automated blood culture systems such as BACTEC definitely enhance the recovery rate of the organism.[3] The median bacterial count of *Salmonella* in the peripheral blood is only 0.3 CFU/mL; hence, sufficient amount of blood should be collected for culture. In adults, at least 10 mL of blood should be collected for culture whereas in children preferably 5 mL blood is to be collected. Dilution of collected blood in the culture media should be appropriate in order to adequately neutralize the bactericidal effect of serum. A ratio of 1:5 to 1:10 of blood to broth is preferred.[1] Clot cultures, where the inhibitory effect of serum is obviated, have not been found to be more sensitive as compared to blood cultures. In the laboratory, blood culture bottles should be incubated at 37° C. They should be checked for turbidity, gas formation, and other evidence of growth after 1, 2, 3 and 7 days. For days 1, 2 and 3 only bottles showing signs of positive growth are cultured on agar plates. On day 7, all bottles should be subcultured before being discarded as culture negative.[1]

There are definite advantages of blood cultures in investigation as they also provide information on the antimicrobial sensitivity of the isolate. A positive culture unequivocally establishes the diagnosis of typhoid.

Bone Marrow Cultures

Salmonella typhi/paratyphi is an intracellular pathogen in the reticuloendothelial cells of the body including the bone marrow. It has been revealed that the median bacteremia in the bone marrow is 9 CFU/mL compared to 0.3 CFU/mL in blood. The bone marrow—peripheral blood ratio which is around 4.8 (IQR 1–27.5) in the first week of illness increases to 158 (IQR 60–397) during the third week owing to disappearance of bacteria from the peripheral blood. The overall sensitivity of bone marrow cultures ranges from 80–95%.[1] Compared to blood culture, it is good even in late disease and despite prior antibiotic therapy.

Bone marrow culture is not considered to be the first line investigation of typhoid fever due to the invasive technique of bone marrow aspiration and some inherent procedural risks albeit minor.[2]

Stool, Urine and Other Cultures

Stool specimen for culture should be collected in a sterile, wide mouthed specimen container. Stool specimens should preferably be processed within 2 hours after sample collection. If delay in processing is anticipated then the specimen should be stored in a refrigerator at 4°C or in a standard cool box with freezer packs. The sensitivity of stool culture depends on the amount of feces sent for culture. The positivity rate increases with the duration of illness. Rectal swabs should be avoided as these are generally less successful. Stool cultures are positive in about 30% of patients with acute typhoid fever.[1] Urine cultures are not usually recommended for diagnosis in view of poor sensitivity.[1] Other methods such as duodenal string and rose snip cultures have been reported to be more efficacious than blood cultures but are mainly of academic importance.

Antimicrobial Sensitivity Testing

Salmonella culture should always be complemented by drug sensitivity testing. Among the various antibiotics used for treatment of typhoid, fluoroquinolones occupy a very significant position. The crucial issue in drug sensitivity testing pertains to fluoroquinolone susceptibility testing.[4] Fluoroquinolones were introduced in clinical use in 1989. Initially, it proved to be very useful but over the last decade there has been a progressive increase in the minimum inhibitory concentrations (MICs) of ciprofloxacin in *S. typhi* and *S. paratyphi*. As a consequence, the use of fluoroquinolones in such scenario is associated with a high incidence of clinical failure. It has been demonstrated that resistance to nalidixic acid is a surrogate marker for high ciprofloxacin MIC's.[5] Thus, it predicts fluoroquinolone failure. Hence, it can be used to select antibiotic therapy. If culture results show resistance to nalidixic acid irrespective of the results of the commonly used fluoroquinolones ciprofloxacin/ofloxacin sensitivity, then fluoroquinolones should not be used. If it has to be used then high doses should be given to overcome the high MIC.[6] Since MIC testing of various antibiotics is not within the scope of most microbiological laboratories, nalidixic acid susceptibility testing is mandatory to help guide choice of antibiotics.[1]

SEROLOGIC TESTS

Widal Test

Widal test is a serological test which detects agglutinating antibodies against O and H antigens of *S. typhi* and *S. paratyphi* A and B.[3] The "O" antigen is the somatic antigen of *S. typhi* and is shared by *S. paratyphi* A and B, and also other *Salmonella* species and other members of the Enterobacteriaceae family. Antibodies against O antigen are predominantly immunoglobulin M (IgM) subtype. The IgM antibody rises early in the illness after the initial exposure to antigen and disappears early. The H antigens are flagellar antigens of *S. typhi*, *S. paratyphi* A and B. Antibodies to H antigens are both IgM and IgG. These antibodies rise late in the illness and persist for a longer time. Usually, O antibodies appear on day 6–8 and H antibodies during days 10–12 after the onset of disease. If the test is performed on an acute serum (at first contact with the patient), then a convalescent serum should preferably also be collected so that paired titrations can be performed.

Ideally, a positive Widal test result implies demonstration of rising titers in paired blood samples at an interval of 10–14 days.[2] But this criterion is purely of academic interest. In practice, decisions about antibiotic therapy cannot wait for results from two samples. Moreover, antibiotics, if administered, may dampen the immune response and as a consequence prevent a rise in titers even in truly infected individuals. Thus, therapeutic decisions have to be generally based on results of a single acute sample test. In typhoid endemic areas, a baseline anti O and anti H antibodies are present in the population owing to repeated subclinical exposure to infections with *S. typhi/paratyphi*, infections with other Enterobacteriaceae, and also other tropical diseases such as dengue and malaria.[1,6]

While interpreting the results of the Widal test, both H and O antibodies have to be considered. There is a controversy about the predictive value of O and H antibodies for diagnosis of typhoid. Some experts claim that O antibodies have superior specificity and positive predictive value (PPV) as these antibodies decline early after an acute infection. On the contrary, other studies report a poorer PPV of O antibodies probably due to rise of these antibodies in other *Salmonella* species or Gram-negative infections, in unrelated infection and following typhoid vaccination.[1,2]

The Widal test as a diagnostic modality has suboptimal sensitivity and specificity. Various studies show that Widal test can be negative in 30% of culture proven cases of typhoid fever. Suboptimal sensitivity also results from negativity in early infection, prior antibiotic therapy, and failure to mount an immune response in some individuals.[1] Poor specificity of Widal test is an even greater problem and it is a consequence of pre-existing baseline antibodies in typhoid endemic areas, cross reactivity with other Gram-negative infections and nontyphoidal *Salmonella* and anamnestic reactions in unrelated infections.[6] The purity and standardization of antigens used for the Widal test is a major factor and often results in poor specificity and poor reproducibility of test results. Widal test done by slide agglutination should also be discouraged, owing to high rate of false positivity.[1,2] For practical purpose, this test should be done after 5–7 days of fever by tube method where levels of both O and H antibodies with 1 in 160 dilution (4-fold rise) or more should be taken as cut-off value for diagnosis.

Other Serologic Tests

Considering the limitations of the Widal test and need for a cheap, easy and rapid diagnostic method, several attempts to develop alternative serologic tests have been made over the years.[1,6] Rapid dipstick assays, dot enzyme immunoassays (EIA), and agglutination inhibition tests are the options.

Enzyme Immunoassay or Typhidot® Test

Typhidot® is a commercially available dot (EIA) that detects IgG and IgM antibodies against a 50 kD outer membrane protein distinct from the somatic (O), flagellar (H), or capsular (Vi) antigen of *S. typhi*.[2] The sensitivity and specificity of this test varies from 70% to 100% and 43% to 90%, respectively. This dot EIA test offers early diagnosis and high negative and positive predictive values (PPVs). Simple method and quick result are the characteristic features of this test. The detection of IgM antibody reveals acute typhoid in the early phase of infection. The detection of both IgG and IgM antibodies suggest acute typhoid in the middle phase of infection. In areas of high endemicity where the rate of typhoid transmission is high, the detection of specific IgG is more common. Since, IgG antibody can persist for more than 2 years after typhoid infection, the detection of specific IgG cannot differentiate between acute and convalescent cases.[6] In addition, false positive results attributable to previous infection may occur. On the other hand, IgG positivity may also occur due to the current reinfection. In cases of reinfection of typhoid, there is a secondary immune response with a significant boosting of IgG over IgM, such that the later cannot be detected and its effect masked. An alternate strategy for solving this problem is to enable the detection of IgM by ensuring that it is unmasked. The original Typhidot® test was modified by inactivating the total IgG in the serum samples. Studies with modified test, Typhidot® M have shown that inactivation of IgG removes competitive binding and allow the access of the antigen to the specific IgM antibody when it is present.[1]

The Typhidot® M that detects only IgM antibodies of *S. typhi* has been reported to be more specific in some studies.

IDL Tubex® Test

The Tubex® test is relatively easy to perform and takes approximately 2 minutes. The test is based on detecting antibodies to a single antigen in *S. typhi* only. The O9 antigen used in this test is very specific and is found in only serogroup D *Salmonella*. A positive Tubex® result always suggests a *Salmonella* infection but does not specify about which group D of *Salmonella* is responsible.[6] Infection by other serotypes like *Salmonella paratyphi* A give negative result. This test detects IgM antibodies but not IgG which is further helpful in the diagnosis of current infections.[1,2]

IgM Dipstick Test

The IgM dipstick test is based on the binding of *S. typhi* specific IgM antibodies to *S. typhi* lipopolysaccharide (LPS) antigen and the staining of the bound antibodies by an antihuman IgM antibody conjugated to colloidal dye particles. This test is beneficial in places where culture facilities are not available.[6] IgM dipstick test can be performed without formal training and in the absence of specialized equipments. It has to be considered that specific antibodies appear a week after the onset of symptoms so the sensitivity of this test increases with time.[1,2]

Antigen Detection Tests

Tests like EIA, counterimmune electrophoresis, and coagglutination to detect serum or urinary somatic/flagellar/Vi antigens of *S. typhi* have been evaluated. Sensitivity of Vi antigen has been found to be superior to somatic and flagellar antigen. The reported sensitivity ranges from 50% to 100% in different studies.[1] Similarly, specificity estimates of the test have been reported to vary from 25% to 90%.[1] The limitations of the Vi antigen detection tests are suboptimal and variable sensitivity and specificity estimates, inability to detect *S. paratyphi* infection/Vi antigen negative strains of *S. typhi*.[6]

MOLECULAR METHODS

The limitations of cultures and serologic tests for typhoid necessitate the development of alternative diagnostic procedures such as polymerase chain reaction (PCR).[2,6] Some patients with culture negative typhoid fever show PCR positivity, suggesting that PCR diagnosis of typhoid may have superior sensitivity than cultures. Over the years some studies have reported PCR methods targeting the flagellin gene, somatic gene, Vi antigen gene, 5S-23S spacer region of the ribosomal RNA gene, invA gene and hilA gene of *S. typhi* for diagnosis of typhoid fever. These studies have reported high sensitivity and specificity when compared to positive blood culture proven and also healthy controls. The turnaround time for diagnosis of typhoid by this method has been less than 24 hours.[1]

There are certain limitations of PCR as follows:[6]

- Clinical utility of PCR tests has not been adequately evaluated
- There exist doubts regarding the interpretation of these tests in individuals with febrile illnesses other than typhoid, those with past history of typhoid, carriers of *S. typhi*, and those vaccinated with typhoid vaccine
- Patients who are clinically diagnosed with typhoid fever and culture negative but PCR positive may in fact be false positives
- Comparison of PCR to the gold standard bone marrow cultures may be a superior method of evaluating the

- PCR tests claim to detect as few as 10 organisms, but in typhoid the median bacteremia is 0.3 CFU/mL of blood. Thus, using small volumes of blood for DNA extraction may significantly lower the sensitivity of these tests
- The high cost and requirement for sophisticated instruments are also potential drawbacks of molecular methods.

CONCLUSION

Complete blood count is the logical and obvious first investigation in febrile children. Presence of a normal or low leukocyte count with eosinopenia in peripheral blood suggests possible typhoid fever.[1,6] It also helps in evaluation and exclusion of alternative diagnoses such as malaria, dengue and other bacteremias. Blood cultures remain the most effective investigation for diagnosis of typhoid till date. Blood culture should be sent early in the course of the illness and most importantly prior to starting antibiotic therapy.[4] Susceptibility testing for nalidixic acid should be routinely done for all isolates to aid the choice and decision of antibiotics.[5,6] Bone marrow culture is a highly sensitive diagnostic test even in late stages of the illness and with prior antibiotic therapy but the fact that it is an invasive procedure prevents its use in routine practice. The Widal test has several limitations and should be requested for in the second week of the illness and its results interpreted with caution. Data on baseline titers in the local population should be generated particularly in endemic region by appropriate studies to help in determining appropriate cut offs for the Widal test. The modified Widal test, Typhidot®, Tubex® and Vi antigen tests need to be evaluated further and as of now they have not been proved to be superior before their routine use can be recommended. Molecular methods are still experimental.

KEY MESSAGES

- Blood cultures remain the gold standard investigation for diagnosis of typhoid. Blood culture should be sent early, prior to starting antibiotic therapy
- Susceptibility testing for nalidixic acid should be routinely done
- Widal test has several limitations and should be requested for in the second week of the illness
- Typhidot, Tubex and Vi antigen tests need to be evaluated further before their routine use can be recommended. Molecular methods are experimental.

REFERENCES

1. Kundu R, Ganguly N, Ghosh TK, et al. IAP Task Force Report: Diagnosis of enteric fever in children. Indian Pediatr 2006;43:875-83.
2. Choudhury J, Kundu R. Enteric fever. In: Choudhury J, Kundu R, editors. Pediatric Infectious Diseases, 1st edition. New Delhi: Jaypee Brothers, 2012;308-20.
3. McKinney JS. Enteric fever (Typhoid fever). In: Kliegman RM, Blum NJ, Shah SS, et al. Nelson Textbook of Pediatrics, 21st edition. Philadelphia: Elsevier, 2020;1502-7.
4. Shastri D, Singhal T. Antimicrobial therapy in enteric fever. In: Singhal T, Shah N, Prabhu S, Yewale V, editors, 3rd edition. New Delhi: Jaypee Brothers, 2019;252-9.
5. Shetty A, Jog S, Rodrigues C. Basic of microbiologic diagnosis. In: Singhal T, Shah N, Prabhu S, Yewale V, editors, 3rd edition. New Delhi: Jaypee Brothers, 2019;3-13.
6. Roy K, Kundu R. Typhoid fever. In: Parthasarathy A, Menon PSN, Nair MKC, et al, editors. IAP Textbook of Pediatrics, 7th edition. New Delhi: Jaypee Brothers, 2019;407-11.

CHAPTER 6

Treatment

INTRODUCTION

In the pre-antibiotic era, typhoid fever was common, complications were frequent and mortality was about 15%. The scenario changed after 1948 when chloramphenicol was discovered. Introduction of chloramphenicol for treatment of typhoid fever resulted in a significant drop in case fatality to 1%. Subsequently, other antibiotics like ampicillin and co-trimoxazole were also effective in treating typhoid. These two antibiotics along with chloramphenicol were the first line drugs used for treatment of typhoid fever for the next 4–5 decades. Nevertheless, these antibiotics were not the ideal as relapses occurred in 5–15% cases and some patients developed chronic carrier stage in gallbladder.

MANAGEMENT

Over the years it has been observed that timely and appropriate treatment and management of typhoid fever can reduce both morbidity and mortality.[1] General supportive measures like use of proper antipyretics, maintenance of adequate hydration, appropriate nutrition and prompt recognition, and early treatment of complications are extremely important for a favorable outcome. The child suffering from typhoid fever should take normal balanced and nutritious diet. Dietary restriction is not required in typhoid fever.[2]

In a typhoid endemic region, 90% or more of typhoid patients can be effectively managed at home. Effective oral antibiotics in appropriate dose and duration along with good nursing care are the mainstay of typhoid management.[3] Close medical follow-up is necessary to look for development of complications or failure to respond to therapy.

The following patients need admission and parenteral antibiotics:[1]
- Patients with persistent vomiting
- Inability to take oral feed
- Severe diarrhea and dehydration
- Abdominal distension.

Antimicrobial Therapy

Since 1990s, *Salmonella typhi* has developed resistance simultaneously to all the drugs used in first line treatment like chloramphenicol, co-trimoxazole and ampicillin in many parts of the world.[2] Resistance to the first line antibiotics is known as Multidrug resistant typhoid fever (MDRTF). *Salmonella* acquired resistance to these first line drugs through R-factor plasmids. Recently, there are some reports of re-emergence of fully susceptible strain to the first line drugs. These reports are not substantiated by proper field studies and hence they are not advocated at present for empirical therapy in typhoid.

Fortunately, by this time fluoroquinolones were available and they proved to be highly efficacious against typhoid fever.[4] They achieved a high cure rate along with fewer relapses and development of chronic gallbladder carrier state. However, following its widespread use in unrelated infections, suboptimal dosing and duration of treatment lead to development of resistance to it within a decade of its use. Fluoroquinolones are not approved by Drug Controller General of India (DCGI) for use under 12 years of age unless the child is resistant to all other recommended antibiotics and is suffering from life-threatening infection.[2]

There is now considerable evidence from the long-term use of fluoroquinolones in children that neither they cause bone or joint toxicity nor do they impair growth. Ciprofloxacin, ofloxacin, pefloxacin, and fleroxacin are common fluoroquinolones proved to be effective and are used in adults for treatment of typhoid fever. In children, the first two are only used in our country and there is no evidence of superiority of any particular fluoroquinolone over others. Fluoroquinolones like ofloxacin or ciprofloxacin are used in a dose of 15 mg/kg/day body weight to a maximum of 20 mg/kg/day. Norfloxacin and nalidixic acid do not achieve adequate blood concentration after oral administration and should not be used.

The resistance to fluoroquinolones may be total or partial. In the laboratory, nalidixic acid resistant *Salmonella typhi* (NARST) is a marker of reduced susceptibility to fluoroquinolones. Resistance to nalidixic acid is a surrogate marker which predicts fluoroquinolones failure and can be used to guide antibiotic therapy.[5]

With the development of fluoroquinolone resistant *S. typhi*, third generation cephalosporins were used in the treatment of typhoid fever. But sporadic reports of resistance to these antibiotics were also noticed from many places.[1] Recently, azithromycin is being used as an alternative drug for treatment of uncomplicated typhoid fever.[2] Aztreonam and imipenem are also potential third line drugs which should ideally be kept in reserve and used when all other antibiotics fail.

Of the third generation cephalosporins, oral cefixime has been widely used in children.[3] Cefixime is used in a dose of

15–20 mg/kg/day in two divided doses. Amongst the third generation injectable cephalosporins, ceftriaxone, cefotaxime and cefoperazone are used of which ceftriaxone is the most convenient. Parenteral dose of ceftriaxone is 60–80 mg/kg/day in one or two divided doses; cefotaxime 100–150 mg/kg/day in two or three doses and cefoperazone 50–100 mg/kg/day in two divided doses. Azithromycin is used in a dose of 20 mg/kg/day in two divided doses.

In uncomplicated typhoid fever, oral third generation cephalosporin, e.g. cefixime should be the drug of choice as empiric therapy.[1] If there is no clinical improvement by 5 days and the culture report is inconclusive, then a second line drug like azithromycin or any other drug effective against *S. typhi* depending upon the sensitivity pattern of that area may be added.[2,5]

For complicated typhoid, the choice of drug is parenteral third generation cephalosporin, e.g. ceftriaxone.[1] In severe life-threatening infection, fluoroquinolones may be used as the last resort. Aztreonam and imipenem may also be used in these situations.

Typhoid fever usually responds to monotherapy. Combination therapy though practiced in some places needs substantiation with adequate data from studies.

Tables 1 and 2 show various antibiotics in the management of both complicated and uncomplicated typhoid with different sensitivity patterns.[1]

There are stray reports of ceftriaxone resistant typhoid fever from different parts of the world. But these were not a major problem as they neither caused any epidemic nor did they lead to widespread affection. In recent times, a large outbreak of multiple drug resistant *S. typhi* has been reported from Sind, Pakistan.[6] These organisms are not only resistant to first line antibiotics like chloramphenicol, ampicillin and co-trimoxa-

TABLE 1

Treatment of uncomplicated typhoid						
Suscepti-bility	First line oral drug			Second line oral drug		
	Antibiotic	Daily Dose (mg/kg)	Days	Antibiotic	Daily Dose (mg/kg)	Days
Fully sensitive	Third generation Cephalosporin e.g. Cefixime	15–20	14	Chloramphenicol	50–75	14–21
				Amoxicillin	100	14
				TMP-SMX	8 TMP 40 SMX	14
Multidrug resistant	Third generation Cephalosporin e.g. Cefixime	15–20	14	Azithromycin	10–20	7

Source: Kundu R, Ganguly N, Ghosh TK, et al. IAP Task Force Report: Management of enteric fever in children. Indian Pediatr 2006;43:884-87, *with permisson.*

zole but also to newer drugs like fluoroquinolones and third generation cephalosporins like ceftriaxone. They carry both plasmid- and chromosome-borne resistance genes to oral first line antibiotics, fluoroquinolones and injectable ceftriaxone.[3] So, the only reliable option left to treat uncomplicated typhoid fever is oral azithromycin and for complicated disease, the injectable carbapenems.[2]

It has been proposed to call these resistant organisms as extensively drug resistant typhoid (XDR typhoid). If they successfully spread worldwide then it will have far reaching consequences. The only treatment option left for serious typhoid is very costly antibiotic carbapenem.

TABLE 2

Treatment of severe typhoid						
Suscep-tibility	First line parenteral drug			Second line parenteral drug		
	Antibiotic	Daily Dose (mg/kg)	Days	Antibiotic	Daily Dose (mg/kg)	Days
Fully sensitive	Ceftriaxone or	60–80	14	Chloramphenicol	100	14–21
	Cefotaxime	100–150		Ampicillin	100	14
				TMP-SMX	8 TMP	
					40 SMX	14
Multidrug resistant	Ceftriaxone or	60–80	14	Aztreonam	50–100	7
	Cefotaxime	100–150				

Note: Imipenem are potential second line drug and fluoroquinolones can be used in life-threatening infection resistant to other recommended antibiotics.

Source: Kundu R, Ganguly N, Ghosh TK, et al. IAP Task Force Report: Management of enteric fever in children. Indian Pediatr 2006;43:884-87, *with permisson.*

ANTIPYRETICS

The aim of fever management is to make the child comfortable and not just bringing down the temperature to normal range. Non-pharmacological management of fever is as important as use of antipyretics. Placing the child in cool airy room, adequate hydration, and mechanical cooling by tepid water sponging often gives much relief.

Antipyretic medicines provide symptomatic relief from the discomfort of elevated body temperature.[2] The most commonly used antipyretic is paracetamol. Paracetamol is generally well tolerated and considered to be the safest antipyretic in children.

Combinations of antipyretics like ibuprofen-paracetamol or mefenamic acid-paracetamol are not indicated.

The most common and preferred route of administration of paracetamol is oral. But paracetamol can be given by rectal suppositories in unconscious patients and in febrile seizure. It can also be given by intravenous (IV) infusion for quick relief.

The dose of paracetamol for oral or suppository in children less than 12 years is 15 mg/kg/dose every 4–6 hourly. In children of age 12–18 years, 325–650 mg every 4–6 hourly. It can be given by IV infusion at 7.5 mg/kg/dose in neonates and infants (maximum 30 mg/kg/day) and 15 mg/kg/dose (maximum 60 mg/kg/day) in older children. The total dose by either route should not exceed 60 mg/kg/day. The antipyretic effect begins within 30–60 minutes and temperature generally reduces by 1–2°C after 2 hours.

TREATMENT OF SEVERE TYPHOID FEVER

Management of hospitalized patients requires:
- Proper use of antibiotics
- Good nursing care
- Adequate nutrition
- Careful attention to fluid and electrolyte balance
- Prompt diagnosis and treatment of complications like intestinal perforation
- Use of high dose of corticosteroids in severely ill patients.

Supportive Measures

Supportive measures are important in the management of severe typhoid fever, such as oral or IV hydration, the use of antipyretics, appropriate nutrition and blood transfusions, if indicated. Also, patients with persistent vomiting, severe diarrhea, and abdominal distension may require hospitalization and parenteral antibiotic therapy.[2]

Steroids in Severe Typhoid Fever

Dexamethasone has been found to reduce the mortality in severe typhoid infection. Typhoid fever patients with changes in mental status should be evaluated for meningitis by examination of the cerebrospinal fluid (CSF). Even if the findings are normal and typhoid meningitis is strongly suspected, children should immediately be treated with high-dose IV dexamethasone in addition to the antimicrobials.[1] Dexamethasone is given in an initial dose of 3 mg/kg by slow IV infusion over 30 minutes followed by 1 mg/kg every 6 hourly for 48 hours. High-dose steroid treatment can be given before the results of typhoid blood cultures are available if other causes of severe disease are unlikely.

Management of Intestinal Perforation

Generalized peritonitis and large amount of pus is seen in patients with perforation of intestine. Appropriate antibiotics, nasogastric suction, resuscitation with IV fluids, blood and oxygen administration are the treatment. If severely toxic, corticosteroids should be given. Antibiotic should cover Gram-negative rods and anaerobes of intestinal flora apart from *Salmonella*. If perforation is confirmed, surgical repair should not be delayed longer than 6 hours. Metronidazole and gentamicin or ceftriaxone should be administered before and after surgery if a fluoroquinolone is not being used to treat leakage of intestinal bacteria into the abdominal cavity.

Management of Intestinal Hemorrhage

Need intensive care monitoring and blood transfusion. Surgical consultation for suspected intestinal perforation is indicated. Most cases of intestinal hemorrhage are not severe and will not require blood transfusion.

Management of Relapse

Relapses involving acute illness have been treated successfully. Cultures should be obtained and standard treatment should be administered. They are sensitive to same antibiotics which were given for the first episode and should be given for a period of 5–7 days.[5]

PROGNOSIS

Factors associated with poor prognosis are:
- Late diagnosis and late initiation of treatment
- Extremes of age (children of less than 2 years and elderly)
- Multidrug resistant (MDR) organism
- Severe disease at the time of presentation
- Associated conditions like HIV infection, sickle cell disease
- Delayed identification of complications
- Delayed initiation of management of complications.

KEY MESSAGES

- ❏ Child suffering from typhoid fever should take normal balanced and nutritious diet
- ❏ Oral third generation cephalosporins like cefixime is effective in the treatment of typhoid fever
- ❏ Azithromycin is being used as an alternative drug for treatment of uncomplicated typhoid fever
- ❏ Patients with persistent vomiting, inability to take oral feed, severe diarrhea, dehydration abdominal distension need admission and parenteral antibiotics
- ❏ For complicated typhoid the choice of drug is parenteral third generation cephalosporin like ceftriaxone

Treatment

- ❑ Combination therapy is not routinely recommended for typhoid fever management
- ❑ Paracetamol is the most commonly used antipyretic, it is well tolerated and considered to be the safest antipyretic in children.

REFERENCES

1. Kundu R, Ganguly N, Ghosh TK, et al. IAP Task Force Report: Management of enteric fever in children. Indian Pediatr 2006;43: 884-87.
2. Choudhury J, Kundu R. Enteric fever. In: Choudhury J, Kundu R, editors. Pediatric Infectious Diseases, 1st edition. New Delhi: Jaypee Brothers, 2012;308-20.
3. Ochoa TJ, Santisteban Ponce J. *Salmonella*. In: Cherry JD, Steinbach WJ, Harrison GJ, Hotez PJ, Kaplan SL, editors. Feigin and Cherry's Textbook of Pediatric Infectious Diseases, 8th edition. Philadelphia: Elsevier, 2019;1066-80.
4. Rodrigues C, Shenai S, Mehta A. Enteric fever in Mumbai, India: The good news and the bad news. Clin Infect Dis 2003;36:535.
5. Shastri D, Singhal T. Antimicrobial therapy in enteric fever. In: Singhal T, Shah N, Prabhu S, Yewale V, editors, 3rd edition. New Delhi: Jaypee Brothers, 2019;252-9.
6. Bhutta ZA, Khan IA, Shadmani M. Failure of short-course ceftriaxone chemotherapy for multidrug-resistant typhoid fever in children: a randomized controlled trial in Pakistan. Antimicrob Agenta Chemother 2000;44:450-2.

CHAPTER 7

Prevention

INTRODUCTION

Typhoid infection is transmitted by ingestion of food or water contaminated with feces containing *Salmonella typhi* or *paratyphi*. So prevention of typhoid is mainly based upon safe water and proper food handling methods.[1]

SAFE WATER

Supply of safe water to the community is of prime importance for prevention of typhoid. Safety of water in not only for drinking but other household requirements like washing, cooking and cleaning.[2]

In urban areas, safe water supply should be ensured from the source to the user. Drinking water should be made available to the public through piped system or via tanker trucks.

In household, safety of water is ensured by boiling, adding chlorine releasing chemicals or exposure to ultraviolet irradiation.

In rural areas, the common sources of water like wells should be checked for pathogens and necessary action should be taken.

Tanks in villages are often important source of water which is subjected to unlimited source of pollution including defecation around the edges. It is used by the poorest in the country without any concept of proper sanitation. This water should not be used as drinking water.

FOOD SANITATION

Contaminated food is also an important source of typhoid.[1,2] Proper hygiene should be implied in the production, handling, distribution and serving of food. Certain important measures include:
- Hands should be scrubbed and washed with soap before food handling and finger nails should be trimmed regularly
- Avoid eating shell fish and raw food without proper disinfection and cooking
- Food should be taken soon after cooking
- Dairy products are notorious for harboring *Salmonella*. It should be stored properly and consumed fresh.

BASIC SANITATION

This will reduce the risk of transmission of *S. typhi* by:
- Proper disposal of human waste thereby imposing a barrier known as sanitation barrier
- Installation and maintenance of sewage treatment plants
- Discouraging the use of human excreta as fertilizer.

HEALTH EDUCATION

Health education and hygiene awareness is one of the most cost effective interventions where vulnerable communities are made aware of the disease and its necessary precaution.[3] This should be inculcated right from the school going children.

> **KEY MESSAGES**
>
> ❏ Prevention of typhoid is mainly based upon safe water and proper food handling methods
> ❏ Health education and hygiene awareness is one of the most cost effective interventions.

REFERENCES

1. Ochoa TJ, Santisteban Ponce J. *Salmonella*. In: Cherry JD, Steinbach WJ, Harrison GJ, Hotez PJ, Kaplan SL, editors. Feigin and Cherry's Textbook of Pediatric Infectious Diseases, 8th edition. Philadelphia: Elsevier, 2019;1066-80.
2. Choudhury J, Kundu R. Enteric fever. In: Choudhury J, Kundu R, editors. Pediatric Infectious Diseases, 1st edition. New Delhi: Jaypee Brothers, 2012;308-20.
3. McKinney JS. Enteric fever (Typhoid fever). In: Kliegman RM, Blum NJ, Shah SS, et al. Nelson Textbook of Pediatrics, 21st edition. Philadelphia: Elsevier, 2020;1502-7.

CHAPTER 8

Vaccines

INTRODUCTION

Typhoid vaccination was part of India's National Immunization Program till 1985. Since then no other typhoid vaccine has been included in the National Immunization Program. A lot of development in typhoid vaccines has taken place and many new typhoid vaccines have been introduced in the market. Considering the endemicity and prevalence of typhoid infection, WHO recommends use of typhoid vaccines in national programs for the control of typhoid fever.

WHOLE CELL INACTIVATED TYPHOID/PARATYPHOID VACCINE

The heat-inactivated phenol-preserved whole-cell typhoid vaccines have been available since the 1890s and they were used extensively in many countries. The vaccine was moderately efficacious (51–88%) in children and young adults in preventing typhoid fever, and the protection persisted for up to 7 years.[1] However, the hindrance was the severe reactogenicity. The incidence of fever was 30% in the vaccinees, headache was up to 10%, and severe local pain was up to 35%. These factors led to the removal from public health programs in most countries.[1]

ORAL INACTIVATED WHOLE CELL VACCINE

The acetone inactivated and formalin inactivated strains of *Salmonella typhi* were used in 1960–1970. They are no longer in use.

NEW-GENERATION TYPHOID VACCINES

The new generation current typhoid vaccines include oral live attenuated Ty21a vaccine, parenteral Vi polysaccharide, and Vi polysaccharide conjugate vaccines.[2] Oral live attenuated Ty21a vaccine is not available in the country, hence will not be discussed in detail.

Live Attenuated Ty21a

Live attenuated Ty21a is formulated as an enteric coated capsule for oral administration. Protection is based on different surface antigens, including O- and H-antigens.[3] A "liquid" formulation that consists of the vaccine in a sachet and buffer in another, which are combined with water before administration, was licensed but it was manufactured only for a short period.[4] The capsules are recommended for individuals aged 5 years and above. In Chile, a study was done on the use of Ty21a typhoid vaccine. Three doses of enteric coated capsule of Ty21a were administered every alternate day. It conferred 67% protection over 3 years and 62% protection over 7 years follow-up. This vaccine was available in India for some time but it is no longer manufactured.

Vi Capsular Polysaccharide Vaccine

The vaccine contains highly purified antigenic fraction of Vi Capsular polysaccharide antigen of *S. typhi* Ty2 strain, which is a virulence factor of the bacteria. It is a linear homopolymer of galacturonic acid purified from the bacteria by treatment with cetavlon. Each dose contains 25 µg of purified polysaccharide in 0.5 mL of phenolic isotonic buffer for intramuscular (IM) use. A single dose of Vi capsular polysaccharide (ViCPS) injectable vaccine provides about 65% protection against blood-culture confirmed typhoid fever for a period of 3 years.[1] The vaccine should be stored at 2–8°C and should not be frozen. The vaccine is stable for 6 months at 37°C and for 2 years at 22°C. Being T-cell independent antigen, it is poorly immunogenic in children below 2 years and is unable to induce booster effect due to poor immunologic memory. Hence, this vaccine is not recommended below 2 years of age.[5]

Efficacy: The biological marker of the vaccine is anti-Vi antibodies and 1 µg/mL is considered as the serologic correlate of protection. It is to be noted that the vaccine does not interfere with the interpretation of Widal test. Efficacy of the vaccine drops over time and the cumulative efficacy at 3 years against culture confirmed typhoid fever is reported to be 55%.[1]

Safety: Side effects are minor. Swelling, pain at the injection site, and fever are observed in some recipients. It can be used in immunocompromised children including those suffering from HIV infection.

The ViCPS vaccine is contraindicated only in those with previous history of hypersensitivity to the vaccine and can be safely given in the immunocompromised children including HIV infected individuals.

Dosage: Typhoid Vi polysaccharide vaccine is recommended for use as a single intramuscular dose in children aged 2 years and above and can safely be given with all other childhood vaccines. Revaccination is recommended every 3 years.[1]

Children suffering from typhoid may be vaccinated 4 weeks after recovery if they have not received the vaccine in preceding 3 years.[6]

Serologic correlates of protection: Unlike many vaccine preventable diseases, serologic correlates of protection are not available for typhoid disease or typhoid vaccines. Hence, even though typically more than 90% of vaccinees achieve seroconversion after unconjugated Vi vaccine, efficacy is actually 50–70% in field efficacy trials.[1]

Vi Capsular Polysaccharide Conjugate Vaccines

The limitations of polysaccharide typhoid vaccines include noneffectiveness below the age of 2 years, limited efficacy (of around 60%), T-cell independent response which lacks immune memory, not boostable, and it does not offer protection against paratyphoid fever. Conjugation of the Vi antigen with a protein carrier is hence desirable as it would induce a T-cell dependent immune response.[5]

The covalent attachment of the polysaccharide to a protein carrier creates a conjugate molecule. This conjugate moiety of the vaccine can convert the T-independent (TI) polysaccharides to T-dependent (TD) by creating an enhanced immune response. Several highly immunogenic proteins have been proposed as the protein component for conjugation. The various conjugation proteins for vaccine production are diphtheria, tetanus toxoid (TT), CRM197, outer membrane protein of *Neisseria meningitidis*, and recombinant *Pseudomonas aeruginosa* exotoxin A (rEPA). The comparison of polysaccharide and conjugate vaccine is shown in Table 1.[1]

TABLE 1

Comparison of polysaccharide and conjugate vaccines	
Polysaccharide vaccine	Conjugate vaccine
T-independent immunogens. Induce mainly IgM/IgG2 (in humans) of low avidity	T-cell dependent immune response to the saccharide, induce higher avidity antibodies
No immunological memory, isotype switching or affinity maturation	Affinity maturation, isotype switching and memory effects
IgM levels drop rapidly: IgG down to 25% after 5 years	Antibody response boosted by repeated immunization
Are not effective in infants under 2 years	Are effective in infants
Immunogenicity depends on molecular weight	Small glycan hapten can make effective vaccine

Vi Capsular Polysaccharide Conjugate Vaccine Conjugated With Pseudomonas aeruginosa Exotoxin A

The US National Institute of Child Health and Disease (NICHD) have developed an improved Vi capsular polysaccharide (ViCPS) conjugate typhoid vaccine. They have used exotoxin A of *Pseudomonas aeruginosa* as a carrier protein. This vaccine candidate subsequently underwent many human clinical trials particularly in Vietnam. The safety and immunogenicity was evaluated initially in adults, then 5- to 14-year-old children and also in 2- to 4-year-old children. None of the recipients experienced high temperature of $>38.5°C$ or significant local reactions after receiving the IM injection.[2]

Vi-polysaccharide Conjugate Vaccine Conjugated with Tetanus Toxoid (5 µg)

There have been efforts to develop a conjugate typhoid vaccine by using different carrier proteins. A conjugate vaccine using tetanus toxoid as the carrier protein was developed in India with a reduced dose of 5 µg of Vi capsular antigen. This vaccine was tested in a clinical trial in 169 subjects with a comparison group (ViCPS) of 37 children >2 years. The results from this study were compared with the NIH study in Vietnam. It was reported that there was 4-fold or greater rise in antibody titer (or an ELISA level higher than the threshold 1 µg/mL) of each group on ELISA which was statistically equivalent to Vi-rEPA. The vaccine was well tolerated with no significant local or systemic side effects. No data on duration of immunity and efficacy of this study was available.[2]

A published school-based cluster randomized trial of 1,765 children, aged 6 months to 12 years with two doses of the vaccine, has demonstrated 100% efficacy of the vaccine in the first year of follow-up with minimum adverse events post vaccination. This is the first efficacy trial of any Vi conjugate typhoid vaccine in India.[2] A subset of these vaccinated cohorts (one dose and two dose groups) was followed up to 30 months post vaccination and no significant advantage of two doses regimen over one dose was noticed.

Vi-polysaccharide Conjugate Vaccine Conjugated with Tetanus Toxoid (25 µg)

Another Vi-capsular polysaccharide conjugate typhoid vaccine conjugated with tetanus toxoid was developed where 25 µg/0.5 mL of conjugate Vi polysaccharide was used.

Phase IIa/IIb study revealed no difference in the geometric mean titers (GMTs) between the two doses (15 µg/0.5 mL) and single (25 µg/0.5 mL) dose cohorts, and a single dose of 25 µg/0.5 mL showed excellent immune response (100% seroconversion). Subsequently a phase III, randomized, multi-centric, controlled trial was conducted. The aim was to evaluate the immunogenicity and safety of this vaccine in a total of 981 healthy subjects. It was compared with the Typhoid Vi capsular polysaccharide vaccine of the same manufacturer having similar amount of antigen per dose.[2]

The study group receiving the test vaccine was divided into two cohorts, i.e. ≥6 months to ≤2 years (327 subjects) and >2 years to <45 years (654 subjects). Cohort I in the study was single arm open label and all the 327 subjects received single dose of the test vaccine. On the other hand, cohort II was randomized, double-blind trial and the subjects were recruited in two groups. One group received a single dose of either test vaccine (340 subjects) and the other received the reference vaccine (314 subjects).

Immunogenicity results: In cohort I of the study, 98.05% subjects showed seroconversion (≥4-fold titer rise) on day 42, and the GMTs on day 0 and 42 were 9.44 U/mL and 1952.03 U/mL respectively. The observed GMTs were slightly higher in >1–2 years than in 6 months to <1 year age group. But there were no difference in seroconversion rates in either of the groups. In cohort II of the study, 97.29% and 93.11% subjects of test and reference vaccine groups respectively, were seroconverted (≥4-fold titer rise) on day 42. The GMTs on day 42 in the test and reference vaccine groups were 1301.44U and 411.11U, respectively (p = 0.00001). Both seroconversion and GMTs were higher in younger (>2 to <15 years) than older (15–45 years) age groups.[2,5]

Long-term immunogenicity: The published 3-year follow-up study demonstrates seroconversion data of Phase III subjects and it shows that GMT of anti-Vi IgG is much higher in the unboostered subgroup following the administration of a single dose of conjugate vaccine as compared to the polysaccharide vaccine.

In the boostered subgroup, GMTs are 3- to 5-fold higher than in unboostered groups at 3 years following a booster dose of conjugate vaccine at 2 years.

IAP ACVIP RECOMMENDATIONS FOR USE

Typhoid conjugate vaccine (TCV) is preferred at all ages as it has improved immunological properties, can be used in younger children, and is expected to provide longer duration of protection.[1,2] It has been observed that approximately 30% of cases of typhoid occur in children below 2 years, and 10% in children aged below 1 year. Considering these factors, WHO has recommended TCV for infants and children from 6 months of age as a 0.5 mL single dose, and the same is endorsed by Indian Academy of Pediatrics (IAP) Advisory Committee on Vaccines and Immunization Practices (ACVIP).

Booster Doses/Revaccination

As per ACVIP, the need for revaccination with typhoid conjugate vaccine is currently unclear. The protection with TCV may last for up to 5 years after the administration of one dose, and natural boosting may occur in endemic areas. Until more data is generated or available, the ACVIP has recommended only a single dose of TCV from 6 months onwards.[2]

If a child has received typhoid polysaccharide vaccine, it is recommended to offer one dose of typhoid conjugate vaccine at least 4 weeks following the receipt of polysaccharide vaccine.[1] Currently, three products of typhoid conjugate vaccine are licensed in India.

Two of them contain 25 μg of purified ViCPS of *S. typhi*, and one of them containing 5 μg purified ViCPS of *S. typhi*. The WHO position paper in 2018 has remarked that the body of evidence for the 5 μg vaccine is very limited.[2]

IAP ACVIP Recommendation on Typhoid Vaccines[2]

Primary Schedule

- A single dose of typhoid conjugate vaccine 25 µg is recommended from the age of 6 months onwards routinely
- An interval of at least 4 weeks is not mandatory between typhoid conjugate vaccine and measles-containing vaccine when it is offered at age of 9 months or beyond
- For a child who has received only typhoid polysaccharide vaccine, a single dose of TCV is recommended at least 4 weeks following the receipt of polysaccharide vaccine. Routine booster for TCV at 2 years is not recommended as of now.

KEY MESSAGES

- Considering the endemicity and prevalence of typhoid infection, WHO recommends routine use of typhoid vaccines
- Use of typhoid polysaccharide vaccine is limited by various factors
- Typhoid conjugate vaccines can be used 6 months onwards
- A single dose of 25 µg typhoid conjugate vaccine has been found to be effective.

REFERENCES

1. Vashishtha VM, Choudhury P, Bansal CP, Yewale VN, Agrawal R. IAP Guidebook on Immunization 2013-14 by Advisory Committee on Vaccination and Immunization Practices (ACVIP). Gwalior: National Publication House, Indian Academy of Pediatrics, 2014.
2. Balasubramanian S, Shah A, Pemde HK, Chatterjee P, et al. Indian Academy of Pediatrics (IAP) Advisory Committee on Vaccines and Immunization Practices (ACVIP) Recommended Immunization

Schedule (2018-19) and Update on Immunization for Children Aged 0 Through 18 Years. Indian Pediatr, 2018;55:1066-74.
3. Indian Academy of Pediatrics Committee on Immunization (IAPCOI). Consensus recommendations on immunization, 2012. Indian Pediatr. 2012;49:550-64.
4. Bhutta ZA, Khan M, Soofi SB, Ochiai L. New Advances in Typhoid Fever Vaccination Strategies, 2011. Adv Experimen Med Biol; 697:17-39. Source: PubMed. Accessed on 27 August 2019.
5. Levine MM. Typhoid fever vaccines. In: Plotkin SA, Orenstein WA, Offit PA, Edwards KM, editors. Plotkin's Vaccines, 7th edition. Philadelphia: Elsevier, 2018;1114-44.
6. Vashistha VM, Kalra A, Thacker N. FAQs on Vaccines & Immunization Practices. New Delhi: Jaypee Brothers Medical Publishers (P) Ltd; 2011.

EU GSPR Authorised Reprsentative
Logos Europe, 9 rue Nicolas Poussin
1700, La Rochelle, France
Phone: +33 (0) 6 67 93 73 78
E-mail: contact@logoseurope.eu

www.ingramcontent.com/pod-product-compliance
Ingram Content Group UK Ltd.
Pitfield, Milton Keynes, MK11 3LW, UK
UKHW021827140426
5217IPUK00016B/1231